Copyright © 2020 by Philips Coleman Ph.d

Table of Contents

Introduction

Cannabis, also known as marijuana, originated in Central Asia but is grown worldwide today. In the United States, it is a controlled substance and is classified as a Schedule I agent (a drug with a high potential for abuse, and no currently accepted medical use). The Cannabis plant produces a resin containing 21-carbon terpenophenolic compounds called cannabinoids, in addition to other compounds found in plants, such as terpenes and flavonoids. The highest concentration of cannabinoids is found in the female flowers of the plant. Delta-9-tetrahydrocannabinol (THC) is the main psychoactive cannabinoid but over 100 other cannabinoids have been reported to be present in the plant. Cannabidiol (CBD) does not produce the characteristic altered consciousness associated with Cannabis but is felt to have potential therapeutic effectiveness and has recently been approved in the form of the pharmaceutical Epidiolex for the treatment of refractory seizure disorders in children. Other cannabinoids that are being investigated for potential medical benefits include cannabinol (CBN), cannabigerol (CBG), and tetrahydrocannabivarin (THCV), although data from human studies are currently unavailable.Clinical trials conducted on medicinal Cannabis are limited. The U.S. Food and Drug Administration (FDA) has not approved the use of Cannabis as a treatment for any medical condition, although both isolated THC and CBD pharmaceuticals are licensed and approved. To conduct clinical drug research with botanical Cannabis in the United States, researchers must file an Investigational New Drug (IND) application with the FDA, obtain a Schedule I license from the U.S. Drug Enforcement Administration, and obtain approval from the National Institute on Drug Abuse.In the 2018 United States Farm Bill, the term hemp is used to describe cultivars of the Cannabis species that contain less than 0.3% THC. Hemp oil or CBD oil are products manufactured from extracts of industrial hemp (i.e., low-THC cannabis cultivars), whereas hemp seed oil is an edible fatty oil that is essentially cannabinoid-free (refer to Table 1). Some products contain other botanical extracts and/or over-the-counter analgesics, and are readily available as oral and topical tinctures or other formulations often advertised for pain management and other purposes. Hemp products containing less than 0.3% of delta-9-THC are not scheduled drugs and could be considered as Farm Bill compliant. Hemp is not a controlled substance; however, CBD is a controlled substance.

History

Cannabis use for medicinal purposes dates back at least 3,000 years.It was introduced into Western medicine in 1839 by W.B. O'Shaughnessy, a surgeon who learned of its medicinal properties while working in India for the British East India Company. Its use was promoted for reported analgesic, sedative, anti-inflammatory, antispasmodic, and anticonvulsant effects.In 1937, the U.S. Treasury Department introduced the Marihuana Tax Act. This Act imposed a levy of $1 per ounce for medicinal use of Cannabis and $100 per ounce for nonmedical use. Physicians in the United States were the principal opponents of the Act. The American Medical Association (AMA) opposed the Act because physicians were required to pay a special tax for prescribing

Cannabis, use special order forms to procure it, and keep special records concerning its professional use. In addition, the AMA believed that objective evidence that Cannabis was harmful was lacking and that passage of the Act would impede further research into its medicinal worth. In 1942, Cannabis was removed from the U.S. Pharmacopoeia because of persistent concerns about its potential to cause harm. Recently, there has been renewed interest in Cannabis by the U.S. Pharmacopeia.In 1951, Congress passed the Boggs Act, which for the first time included Cannabis with narcotic drugs. In 1970, with the passage of the Controlled Substances Act, marijuana was classified by Congress as a Schedule I drug. Drugs in Schedule I are distinguished as having no currently accepted medicinal use in the United States. Other Schedule I substances include heroin, LSD, mescaline, and methaqualone.Despite its designation as having no medicinal use, Cannabis was distributed by the U.S. government to patients on a case-by-case basis under the Compassionate Use Investigational New Drug program established in 1978. Distribution of Cannabis through this program was closed to new patients in 1992. Although federal law prohibits the use of Cannabis, Figure 1 below shows the states and territories that have legalized Cannabis use for medical purposes. Additional states have legalized only one ingredient in Cannabis, such as cannabidiol (CBD), and are not included in the map. Some medical marijuana laws are broader than others, and there is state-to-state variation in the types of medical conditions for which treatment is allowed.The main psychoactive constituent of Cannabis was identified as delta-9-tetrahydrocannabinol (THC). In 1986, an isomer of synthetic delta-9-THC in sesame oil was licensed and approved for the treatment of chemotherapy-associated nausea and vomiting under the generic name dronabinol. Clinical trials determined that dronabinol was as effective as or better than other antiemetic agents available at the time. Dronabinol was also studied for its ability to stimulate weight gain in patients with AIDS in the late 1980s. Thus, the indications were expanded to include treatment of anorexia associated with human immunodeficiency virus infection in 1992. Clinical trial results showed no statistically significant weight gain, although patients reported an improvement in appetite. Another important cannabinoid found in Cannabis is CBD. This is a nonpsychoactive cannabinoid, which is an analog of THC.In recent decades, the neurobiology of cannabinoids has been analyzed. The first cannabinoid receptor, CB1, was identified in the brain in 1988. A second cannabinoid receptor, CB2, was identified in 1993. The highest expression of CB2 receptors is located on B lymphocytes and natural killer cells, suggesting a possible role in immunity. Endogenous cannabinoids (endocannabinoids) have been identified and appear to have a role in pain modulation, control of movement, feeding behavior, mood, bone growth, inflammation, neuroprotection, and memory.Nabiximols (Sativex), a Cannabis extract with a 1:1 ratio of THC:CBD, is approved in Canada (under the Notice of Compliance with Conditions) for symptomatic relief of pain in advanced cancer and multiple sclerosis. Nabiximols is an herbal preparation containing a defined quantity of specific cannabinoids formulated for oromucosal spray administration with potential analgesic activity. Nabiximols contains extracts from two Cannabis plant varieties. The extracts mixture is standardized to the concentrations of the psychoactive delta-9-THC and the nonpsychoactive CBD. The preparation also contains other, more minor cannabinoids, flavonoids, and terpenoids. Canada,

New Zealand, and most countries in western Europe also approve nabiximols for spasticity of multiple sclerosis, a common symptom that may include muscle stiffness, reduced mobility, and pain, and for which existing therapy is unsatisfactory.

What is CBD?

CBD is 1 of the hundreds of chemicals found in the flowering cannabis plant. CBD does not have the psychoactive, or mind-altering, effects of another chemical found in cannabis called tetrahydrocannabinol (THC). THC is the chemical that causes people to experience a "high." CBD, on the other hand, is being used by some to help ease pain, anxiety, and sleep issues. CBD comes from cannabis plants called hemp that are specifically grown with high levels of CBD and low levels of THC. Cannabis plants grown with high levels of THC are usually called marijuana. CBD comes from oil that is extracted from the cannabis plant. That oil can then be ingested as a liquid, a capsule, a gummy, or inhaled through vaping. It can also be added as an ingredient in such products as lotions and skin patches.

What is cannabis?

Cannabis refers to a group of three plants with psychoactive properties, known as Cannabis sativa, Cannabis indica, and Cannabis ruderalis. When the flowers of these plants are harvested and dried, you're left with one of the most common drugs in the world. Some call it weed, some call it pot, and others call it marijuana. As weed becomes legal in more areas, names for it are evolving. Today, more and more people are using the term cannabis to refer to weed. Some argue that it's a more accurate name. Others feel it's more neutral compared with terms like weed or pot, which some people associate with its illegal use. Also, the term "marijuana" is falling out of favor due to its racist history. Cannabis is usually consumed for its relaxing and calming effects. In some U.S. states, it's also prescribed to help with a range of medical conditions, including chronic pain, glaucoma, and poor appetite. Keep in mind that while cannabis comes from a plant and is considered natural, it can still have strong effects, both positive and negative.

Types of cannabis

Cannabis Sativa

Sativa is the marijuana type that people seem to like smoking the most. This plant grows quite large, reaching up to 15 feet in some cases. While it is not a really thick plant, many growers like it due to how tall it can grow.Their leaves are long, dainty, narrow, and considering their height potential, these are perfect for outdoor growing. The seeds are soft to the touch, with no spots or markings on them. Do not expect this plant to flower quickly because Sativa takes its precious time, and even shifting the light cycles could have little effect on this.Sativa is usually found below a latitude of 30° N, in places like India, Thailand, Nigeria, Mexico, and Colombia. Sativa is often dried, cooked and consumed. While many people either vaporize or smoke this strain, it is the norm for users to use this to get high.It also can enhance your creativity, depending on the person. This is the strain you use when you want to be up and active during the day since it raises your energy and opens you up to fresh, new ideas. If you are an artist of some sort, you may love this one. Sativa is known for a high ratio of THC to CBN the two primary active ingredients in cannabis. Sativa dominant strains are higher in the THC cannabinoid. This makes it less likely to be used for medicinal purposes, but it is still common in Ayurvedic medicine.

They also work well to combat the symptoms of:

- Depression
- ADHD
- Fatigue
- Mood disorders
- Growing Cannabis Sativa

Cannabis Sativa is a type of marijuana that typically flowers for longer, has lower yields than Cannabis Indica, and has characteristically long thin leaves. They're taller plants in general since they come from a region near the equator, which has longer summers (which is also why their flowering period naturally lasts longer). A good thing about growing Cannabis Sativa is that the vegetative phase is shorter. There are even some Sativas out there bred to have shorter flowering phases. If you're from a hotter climate or have trouble keeping your grow room temperatures down, then a Sativa might be for you — they can take high temperatures better than Indicas.

Cannabis Indica

Cannabis Indica is a more solid strain in comparison to Sativa, but it does not have the height Sativa achieves. Indica strains generally grow between 3 to 6 feet tall (1 to 2 meters. It is a bushy plant with round healthy leaves, unlike Sativa. However, they both have marbled colored, soft seeds. Being that Indica is a short plant, this one is perfect for indoor growing.While Sativa takes some time to flower, Indica flowers much faster and can be influenced a lot easier by adjusting the light cycle to promote this

phase. It is most commonly found above 30° N, in countries like Nepal, Lebanon, Morocco, and Afghanistan. The buds and flowers on Indica dominant strains will usually grow very close to each other and are stickier to the touch than Sativa plants. When you want to make hashish, Indica is the plant you would choose due to the amount of resin it contains.

Cannabis Indica has lovely healing qualities, and helps with:

- Insomnia
- Alleviating pain
- Inducing relaxation of muscles
- Muscle spasms
- Calming anxiety
- Headache and migraine relief

Growing Cannabis Indica

Cannabis Indica is a strain of medical marijuana that is typically higher yielding, has a shorter flowering time, and has leaves that are shorter and wider than a

Sativa's. They're smaller plants in general, but they can get quite bushy. Lots of growers prefer growing Indicas for these reasons. Because of their shorter flowering phase, people who grow in colder climates with shorter winters may want to grow Indicas. Because of their shorter height, growing them indoors is also easy when it comes to growing Indicas.

Cannabis Ruderalis

You will rarely hear anyone talking about Cannabis Ruderalis, which is one of the primary marijuana types and has a pretty short stature growing between 20-25 inches in height. Similar to Indica, this plant has very thick foliage. This plant is usually found growing in northern regions of the world.Ruderalis has an extremely early and fast flowering cycle because it grows farther north than any other type of marijuana and so doesn't have the luxury of a lot of time to mature before cold weather hits. Ruderalis is used to produce autoflowerers. One of the reasons you hear little about this strain is because it is not known to be highly psychotropic. It is used primarily as a source of additional genetic material by breeders and cultivators. That way, hybrids which flower early can be bred, and certain strains can be adjusted so that they will grow in more northerly climates.

Industrial hemp marijuana types

Industrial hemp or hemp, typically found in the northern hemisphere, is a type of marijuana originating from the Cannabis Sativa species that is grown specifically for the industrial uses of its derived products.

It is one of the fastest growing plants and was one of the first plants to be spun into usable fiber 10,000 years ago. It can be refined into a variety of commercial items including paper, textiles, clothing, biodegradable plastics, paint, insulation, biofuel, food, and animal feed.Hemp was a cash crop in America until the passage of the 1937 Marihuana Tax Act, partially because hemp can grow wild in climates where winter doesn't freeze the soil and kill the seeds. According to the USDA, hemp has a low THC content and isn't worth smoking. With THC levels below 0,3%, I totally agree.

Hybrid marijuana types

In modern cannabis cultivation and breeding, there are a huge number of varieties available. Many years of intense mixing and hybridization have created a huge spectrum across these three primary varieties.The different mixes all have different characteristics, running the gamut of possibilities relating to flowering cycles, yield, CBN:THC ratios, and disease resistance, among others. In general, the purpose of a hybrid plant is to combine positive characteristics from different strains together. Some key differences between Indica and Sativa marijuana types are the height of the plants, the length between buds, the size and shape of the leaves, the odor, the quality of the smoke, and the chemical properties themselves. In general,

Indica is wide and robust while Sativa is long and thin.

Growing Hybrids

Hybrids can vary greatly, but usually, they have some of the good qualities of both Sativas and Indicas. Because of the range of genes you can find in hybrid marijuana plants, it's hard to specify a common height, leaf shape, or other distinguishing detail. However, hybrids are often bred to have higher yields and be more pest-resistant, which is great for growers. Hybrids are extremely popular. Most of the seeds available are hybrids. To know what you can expect, be sure to read the growth descriptions before buying.

Male cannabis plants

When male-sexed cannabis plants finish maturing, the flowering process occurs all across the plant. Tiny racemes (short flower stalks) are formed at the base of the flower itself. When the flowers open, the plant releases a load of airborne pollen which sticks to and is absorbed by the pistil of the female plant. This is a basic explanation of how the fertilization and reproductive process in cannabis plants works. It can be difficult to distinguish between male and female plants at times, but the male usually has earlier sexual development.

Female cannabis plants

Like male cannabis plants, mature females will also produce racemes. In the case of the female plants, the racemes are a blend of tiny pistils and calyces (calyx). In each of the calyces, there is an ovule, which acts as the receptor for the pollen from the male plant. When the grains of pollen stick to a pistil, the pistil stalk then pushes into the calyx, and the plant is fertilized. The calyx itself is also the site where cannabis seeds are grown after fertilization. Each seed will have a mix of characteristics coming from both parent plants, as in other instances of sexual reproduction. The only time this wouldn't be the case would be if

the parent plants were identical, as in the case of certain pure clones or specific hybridizations.

Hermaphrodite cannabis plants

Although rare as a natural occurrence in nature, many growers might be exposed to the existence of hermaphroditic plants, that is, plants that contain both male and female sex organs. These sorts of plants can fertilize themselves, which is both extremely interesting and potentially quite useful from a breeding perspective. In general, a hermaphrodite cannabis plantfalls on one of the three points along a sexual spectrum. If the plant is mainly comprised of male flowers or has a roughly equal number of male/female flowers, it is probably of little use to a grower. If the hermaphrodite has mainly female flowers, however, it should definitely be saved. The pollen from these plants can be quite useful, and some growers collect the pollen because even though it is a male part of reproduction, the hermaphroditic pollen is genetically female, and will produce female flowers. In the '70s, Indica strains were brought to the USA and mixed with the already present Sativa plants, which set off a long chain of breeding and experimentation with cannabis cultivation and hybridization.It's important to note that despite the differences between all of these types of marijuana, they are essentially one species. They can still be bred together. The names Indica and Sativa refer to the areas where the plants are originally from. The same sort of idea is found in other agriculture, or dog breeds, where there is a wide difference in appearances, but the species are still the same.

What Is Cancer?

Cancer is the name given to a collection of related diseases. In all types of cancer, some of the body's cells begin to divide without stopping and spread into surrounding tissues.Cancer can start almost anywhere in the human body, which is made up of trillions of cells. Normally, human cells grow and divide to form new cells as the body needs them. When cells grow old or become damaged, they die, and new cells take their place.When cancer develops, however, this orderly process breaks down. As cells become more and more abnormal, old or damaged cells survive when they should die, and new cells form when they are not needed. These extra cells can divide without stopping and may form growths called tumors.Many

cancers form solid tumors, which
are masses of tissue. Cancers of
the blood, such as leukemias,
generally do not form solid
tumors.Cancerous tumors are
malignant, which means they can
spread into, or invade, nearby
tissues. In addition, as these
tumors grow, some cancer cells
can break off and travel to distant
places in the body through the
blood or the lymph system and
form new tumors far from the
original tumor.Unlike malignant
tumors, benign tumors do not
spread into, or invade, nearby

tissues. Benign tumors can sometimes be quite large, however. When removed, they usually don't grow back, whereas malignant tumors sometimes do. Unlike most benign tumors elsewhere in the body, benign brain tumors can be life threatening.

What causes cancer?

You would not believe how many emails we get from cancer patients who have gone through these three steps:

- The patient had chemotherapy, radiation, and surgery to treat their cancer;
- The patient was told they were "cancer-free";
- Months later cancer "came back," which is called "regression."

- Among other things, this article will explain what went wrong and how to prevent cancer from coming back. When talking about what causes cancer we need to talk about it at two different levels.
- The first level is talking about cancer at the systemic level, meaning what conditions in the body allowed cancer to grow out of control and how do we deal with this issue.
- The second level of talking about cancer is talking about what causes cancer at the

cellular level. In other words, why does a healthy cell become cancerous?

Understanding your cancer

Picking a single cancer treatment, any single treatment, is the most common mistake made by cancer patients who are new to alternative medicine. Many alternative cancer treatments can be combined.

Dr. Patrick Quillin contends cancer patients should focus on the parts of the body that are working properly, not on cancer.

He suggests a 21-day path to health, noting nutrients from food and supplements change the way your body works, making it less receptive to cancer cells and more supportive of healthy cells.

Dr. Quillin points out it is important to understand how cancer starts and progresses in the human body

including through malnutrition.
Primary causes of cancer include:

poor nutrition — an excess,
deficiency, or imbalance of any
nutrients;

stress — the mind generates
chemicals that can lower
protective mechanisms against
cancer;

sedentary lifestyle — exercise
helps to oxygenate and regulate
the entire body;

toxic burden — hence
detoxification becomes crucial.

Differences between Cancer Cells and Normal Cells

Cancer cells differ from normal cells in many ways that allow them to grow out of control and become invasive. One important difference is that cancer cells are less specialized than normal cells. That is, whereas normal cells mature into very distinct cell types with specific functions, cancer cells do not. This is one reason that, unlike normal cells, cancer cells continue to divide without stopping.In addition, cancer cells are able to ignore signals that normally tell cells to stop dividing or that begin a process known as programmed cell death, or apoptosis, which the body uses to get rid of unneeded cells.Cancer cells may be able to influence the normal cells, molecules, and blood vessels that surround and feed a tumor—an area known as the microenvironment. For instance, cancer cells can induce nearby normal cells to form blood vessels that supply tumors with oxygen and nutrients, which they need to grow. These blood vessels also remove waste products from tumors. Cancer cells are also often able to evade the immune system, a network of organs, tissues, and specialized cells that protects the body from infections and other conditions. Although the immune system normally removes damaged or abnormal cells from the body, some cancer cells are able to "hide" from the immune system.Tumors can also use the immune system to stay alive and grow. For example, with the help of certain immune system cells that normally prevent a runaway immune response, cancer cells can actually keep the immune system from killing cancer cells.

How Cancer Arises

Genetic changes that cause cancer can be inherited from our parents. They can also arise during a person's lifetime as a result of errors that occur as cells divide or because of damage to DNA caused by certain environmental exposures. Cancer-causing environmental exposures include substances, such as the chemicals in tobacco smoke, and radiation, such as ultraviolet rays from the sun. (Our Cancer Causes and Prevention section has more information.)Each person's cancer has a unique combination of genetic changes. As the cancer continues to grow, additional changes will occur. Even within the same tumor, different cells may have different genetic changes.In general, cancer cells have more genetic changes,

such as mutations in DNA, than normal cells. Some of these

changes may have nothing to do with the cancer; they may be the result of the cancer, rather than its cause.

"Drivers" of Cancer

The genetic changes that contribute to cancer tend to affect three main types of genes—proto-oncogenes, tumor suppressor genes, and DNA repair genes. These changes are sometimes called "drivers" of cancer.Proto-oncogenes are involved in normal cell growth and division. However, when these genes are altered in certain ways or are more active than normal, they may become cancer-causing genes (or oncogenes), allowing cells to grow and survive when they should not. Tumor suppressor genes are also involved in controlling cell growth and division. Cells with certain alterations in tumor suppressor genes may divide in an uncontrolled manner.DNA repair genes are involved in fixing damaged DNA. Cells with mutations in these genes tend to develop additional mutations in other genes. Together, these mutations may cause the cells to become cancerous.As scientists have learned more about the molecular changes that lead to cancer, they have found that certain mutations commonly occur in many types of cancer. Because of this, cancers are sometimes characterized by the types of genetic alterations that are believed to be driving them, not just by where they develop in the body and how the cancer cells look under the microscope.

When Cancer Spreads

A cancer that has spread from the place where it first started to another place in the body is called metastatic cancer. The process by which cancer cells spread to other parts of the body is called metastasis.Metastatic cancer has the same name and the same type of cancer cells as the original, or primary, cancer. For example, breast cancer that spreads to and forms a metastatic tumor in the lung is metastatic breast cancer, not lung cancer.Under a microscope, metastatic cancer cells generally look the same as cells of the original cancer. Moreover, metastatic cancer cells and cells of the original cancer usually have some molecular features in common, such as the presence of specific chromosome changes. Treatment may help prolong the lives of some people with metastatic cancer. In general, though, the primary goal of treatments for metastatic cancer is to control the growth of the cancer or to relieve symptoms caused by it. Metastatic tumors can cause severe damage to how the body functions, and most people who die of cancer die of metastatic disease.

Tissue Changes that Are Not Cancer

Not every change in the body's tissues is cancer. Some tissue changes may develop into cancer if they are not treated, however. Here are some examples of tissue changes that are not cancer but, in some cases, are monitored:

Hyperplasia occurs when cells within a tissue divide faster than normal and extra cells build up, or proliferate. However, the cells and the way the tissue is organized look normal under a microscope. Hyperplasia can be caused by several factors or conditions, including chronic irritation.

Dysplasia is a more serious condition than hyperplasia. In dysplasia, there is also a buildup of extra cells. But the cells look abnormal and there are changes in how the tissue is organized. In general, the more abnormal the cells and tissue look, the greater the chance that cancer will form.

Some types of dysplasia may need to be monitored or treated. An example of dysplasia is an abnormal mole (called a dysplastic nevus) that forms on the skin. A dysplastic nevus can turn into melanoma, although most do not.

An even more serious condition is carcinoma in situ. Although it is sometimes called cancer, carcinoma in situ is not cancer because the abnormal cells do not spread beyond the original tissue. That is, they do not invade nearby tissue the way that cancer cells do. But, because some carcinomas in situ may become cancer, they are usually treated.

Types of Cancer

There are more than 100 types of cancer. Types of cancer are usually named for the organs or tissues where the cancers form. For example, lung cancer starts in cells of the lung, and brain cancer starts in cells of the brain. Cancers also may be described by the type of cell that formed them, such as an epithelial cell or a squamous cell. You can search NCI's website for information on specific types of cancer based on the cancer's location in the body or by using our A to Z List of Cancers. We also have collections of information on childhood cancers and cancers in adolescents and young adults.

Here are some categories of cancers that begin in specific types of cells:

Carcinoma

Carcinomas are the most common type of cancer. They are formed by epithelial cells, which are the cells that cover the inside and outside surfaces of the body. There are many types of epithelial cells, which often have a column-like shape when viewed under a microscope.

Carcinomas that begin in different epithelial cell types have specific names:

Adenocarcinoma is a cancer that forms in epithelial cells that produce fluids or mucus. Tissues with this type of epithelial cell are sometimes called glandular tissues. Most cancers of the breast, colon, and prostate are adenocarcinomas.

Basal cell carcinoma is a cancer that begins in the lower or basal (base) layer of the epidermis, which is a person's outer layer of skin.

Squamous cell carcinoma is a cancer that forms in squamous cells, which are epithelial cells that lie just beneath the outer surface of the skin. Squamous cells also line many other organs, including the stomach, intestines, lungs, bladder, and kidneys. Squamous cells look flat, like fish scales, when viewed under a microscope. Squamous cell carcinomas are sometimes called epidermoid carcinomas.

Transitional cell carcinoma is a cancer that forms in a type of epithelial tissue called transitional epithelium, or urothelium. This tissue, which is made up of many layers of epithelial cells that can get bigger and smaller, is found in the linings of the bladder, ureters, and part of the kidneys (renal pelvis), and a few other organs. Some cancers of the bladder, ureters, and kidneys are transitional cell carcinomas.

Sarcoma

Osteosarcoma is the most common cancer of bone. The most common types of soft tissue sarcoma are leiomyosarcoma, Kaposi sarcoma, malignant fibrous histiocytoma, liposarcoma, and dermatofibrosarcoma protuberans.

Leukemia

Cancers that begin in the blood-forming tissue of the bone marrow are called leukemias. These cancers do not form solid tumors.

Instead, large numbers of abnormal white blood cells (leukemia cells and leukemic blast cells) build up in the blood and bone marrow, crowding out normal blood cells. The low level of normal blood cells can make it harder for the body to get oxygen to its tissues, control bleeding, or fight infections. There are four common types of leukemia, which are grouped based on how quickly the disease gets worse (acute or chronic) and on the type of blood cell the cancer starts in (lymphoblastic or myeloid).

Lymphoma

Lymphoma is cancer that begins in lymphocytes (T cells or B cells). These are disease-fighting white blood cells that are part of the immune system. In lymphoma, abnormal lymphocytes build up in lymph nodes and lymph vessels, as well as in other organs of the body.

There are two main types of lymphoma:

Hodgkin lymphoma – People with this disease have abnormal lymphocytes that are called Reed-

Sternberg cells. These cells usually form from B cells.

Non-Hodgkin lymphoma – This is a large group of cancers that start in lymphocytes. The cancers can grow quickly or slowly and can form from B cells or T cells.

Multiple Myeloma

Multiple myeloma is cancer that begins in plasma cells, another type of immune cell. The abnormal plasma cells, called myeloma cells, build up in the bone marrow and form tumors in bones all through the body. Multiple myeloma is also called plasma cell myeloma and Kahler disease.

Melanoma

Melanoma is cancer that begins in cells that become melanocytes, which are specialized cells that make melanin (the pigment that gives skin its color). Most melanomas form on the skin, but melanomas can also form in other pigmented tissues, such as the eye.

Brain and Spinal Cord Tumors

There are different types of brain and spinal cord tumors. These tumors are named based on the type of cell in which they formed and where the tumor first formed in the central nervous system. For example, an astrocytic tumor begins in star-shaped brain cells called astrocytes, which help keep nerve cells healthy. Brain tumors can be benign (not cancer) or malignant (cancer).

Other Types of Tumors

Germ Cell Tumors

Germ cell tumors are a type of tumor that begins in the cells that give rise to sperm or eggs. These tumors can occur almost anywhere in the body and can be either benign or malignant.

Neuroendocrine Tumors

Neuroendocrine tumors form from cells that release hormones into the blood in response to a signal from the nervous system. These tumors, which may make higher-than-normal amounts of hormones, can cause many different symptoms. Neuroendocrine tumors may be benign or malignant.

Carcinoid Tumors

Carcinoid tumors are a type of neuroendocrine tumor. They are slow-growing tumors that are usually found in the gastrointestinal system (most often in the rectum and small intestine). Carcinoid tumors may spread to the liver or other sites in the body, and they may secrete substances such as serotonin or prostaglandins, causing carcinoid syndrome.

Can CBD help people with cancer?

Studies to answer this question are underway. Some scientists are studying whether CBD could relieve some of the side effects of cancer and its treatment, such as pain, insomnia, anxiety, or nausea. Other scientists are studying whether CBD could potentially slow or stop the growth of cancer.To date, no large-scale studies have shown CBD to have benefits for the treatment of people with cancer. Most studies that have been done evaluating CBD as a cancer treatment were in mice or in human cells in the lab. For instance, there are some studies that have shown that CBD inhibits the growth of cancer cells in mice with lung cancer or colon cancer. Another study showed that CBD, together with THC, killed glioblastoma cancer cells in the lab. However, no studies have been conducted in people with cancer.There have been some studies that show that CBD, alone or together with THC, may relieve pain, insomnia, or anxiety, but these studies were not specific to people with cancer. While no studies to date have shown that CBD eases these side effects specifically in people with cancer or people receiving cancer treatment, some people with cancer have reported benefits in taking CBD, such as helping with nausea, vomiting, depression, and other side effects. According to

ASCO guidelines, your doctor may consider prescribing cannabinoids for chronic pain management if you live in a state where it is legal. However, ASCO guidelines state that there is not enough evidence to support the use of cannabinoids for preventing nausea and vomiting in people with cancer receiving radiation therapy or chemotherapy.There are 2 synthetic cannabis medications, nabilone (Cesamet) and dronabinol (Marinol or Syndros), that are FDA-approved to treat nausea and vomiting related to chemotherapy.

These medications are made in a laboratory.

Is CBD safe for people with cancer?

You may find stories online of people discussing the benefits of CBD as a cancer treatment or as relief for side effects. Please remember that such personal stories, while they may be well-meaning, are shared without scientific study and do not constitute evidence. The safety and efficacy of CBD for people with cancer still has to be proven in large, randomized, controlled clinical trials. It is also important to note that some studies have shown that CBD might interfere with how your body processes cancer drugs, called a drug interaction. This might make cancer treatments more toxic or make them less effective. More research is needed on these effects, too. For these reasons, always tell your oncologist if you're thinking about using CBD before you take it.You may also be wondering if CBD is legal in your area. Some states allow the sale and possession of cannabis, including CBD and THC, for medical and recreational use. Others have stricter regulations, so state-by-state laws should always be learned before transporting CBD across state lines. Things are more complicated at the federal level. In 2018, the U.S. government recognized that hemp can be grown and manufactured legally as part of the Farm Act. Hemp can be used to make things like rope and clothing, in addition to CBD oil. In other words, hemp is no longer a controlled substance, which means it is not regulated by the government. This means that consumers have to evaluate the safety and quality of CBD products on their own. Some CBD, for example, may have much higher levels of THC than what is labeled. The bottom line is this: Always talk to your doctor first if you're thinking about using CBD. Because the research does not yet support the use of CBD in helping people with cancer, it's important to raise the topic with your doctor before taking it. There are several clinical trials underway studying the use of CBD in cancer care, and you and your oncologist can talk through the possible benefits and risks of you joining a research study to help find answers to some of the questions about CBD, including whether it may reduce side effects or improve quality of life.

As a treatment for cancer

There's solid evidence supporting the idea that cannabinoids can reduce tumor growth in animal models of cancer. CBD may also enhance uptake or increase the potencyTrusted Source of certain drugs used to treat cancer.

Here are some promising studies:

A 2019 review of in vitro and in vivo studies focusing on pancreatic cancer found that cannabinoids can help slow tumor growth, reduce tumor invasion, and induce tumor cell death. The study authors wrote that research into the effectiveness of different formulations, dosing, and precise mode of action is lacking and urgently needed.

A 2019 studyTrusted Source indicated that CBD could provoke cell death and make glioblastoma cells more sensitive to radiation, but with no effect on healthy cells.A large, long-term study of men within the California Men's Health Study cohort found that using cannabis may be inversely associated with bladder cancer risk. However, a cause and effect relationship hasn't been established.A 2014 study in experimental models of colon cancer in vivo suggests that CBD may inhibit the spread of colorectal cancer cells.A 2014 review of 35 in vitro and in vivo studies found that cannabinoids are promising compounds in the treatment of gliomas.Research from 2010 demonstrated the efficacy of CBD in preclinical models of metastatic breast cancer. The study found that CBD significantly reduced breast cancer cell proliferation and invasion. These are just a few studies addressing the potential of cannabinoids to help treat cancer. Still, it's far too soon to say that CBD is a safe and effective treatment for cancer in humans. CBD shouldn't be considered a substitute for other cancer treatments.

Some areas for future research include:

- the effects of CBD with and without other cannabinoids like THC

- safe and effective dosing
- the effects of different administration techniques
- how CBD works on specific types of cancer
- how CBD interacts with chemotherapy drugs and other cancer treatments

As a complementary treatment for cancer

Cancer treatments such as chemotherapy and radiation can produce an array of side effects, such as nausea and loss of appetite, which can lead to weight loss.Research suggests that cannabinoids may ease neuropathic pain and nausea. THC has shown to improve poor appetite due to cancer and cancer treatment, while CBD can suppress it. CBD is also thoughtTrusted Source to have anti-inflammatory and anti-anxiety properties.So far, only one CBD product has received Food and Drug Administration (FDA) approval.That product is Epidiolex, and its only use is in the treatment of two rare forms of epilepsy. No CBD products have been FDA-approved to treat cancer or symptoms of cancer, or to ease side effects of cancer treatment. On the other hand, two synthetic THC drugs have been approved to treat nausea and vomiting caused by chemotherapy. Dronabinol comes in a capsule (Marinol) and tincture form (Syndros) and contains THC. Nabilone (Cesamet) is an oral synthetic cannabinoid that acts similar to THC. Another cannabinoid drug, nabiximols, is available in Canada and parts of Europe. It's a mouth spray containing both THC and CBD and has shown promise in treating cancer pain. It's not approved in the United States, but it is the subject of ongoing research. If you're considering using medical marijuana, talk to your doctor about how best to administer it. Smoking may not be a good choice for people with certain types of cancer.CBD and other cannabis products come in many forms, including vape, tincture, sprays, and oils. They can also be found in candies, coffee, or other edibles.

CANNABIS FOR CANCER SYMPTOMS & CHEMOTHERAPY SIDE EFFECTS

Dr. Dustin Sulak is an integrative osteopathic physician and medical cannabis expert whose clinical practice has focused on treating refractory conditions in adults and children since 2009. He is the founder of Integr8 Health, with offices in Maine, that follows more than 8,000 patients using medical cannabis and other integrative healing modalities. Sulak has published in the peer-reviewed literature, and lectures to health-care providers internationally on the clinical applications of cannabis. The following information is adapted, with permission, from Sulak's educational website, Healer.com, which offers a range of programs about medical cannabis, as well as medical cannabis training and a certification program for physicians, other health professionals, and consumers.When working with cancer patients, cannabis treatment efforts often take two distinct paths — using cannabis to reduce symptoms and improve treatment tolerability, or using cannabis, typically in high doses, to help kill the cancer. The goals aren't mutually exclusive, according to Sulak, but each requires a different approach to dosing.When used properly, cannabis can be a safe, effective treatment for cancer patients with chronic pain, insomnia, and chemotherapy-induced nausea and vomiting. Animal studies have shown that cannabinoids can prevent the development of neuropathic pain, a common chemotherapy side effect that can limit a patient's chemo dose or course. Even after achieving cancer remission, many patients are left with debilitating neuropathic pain that can be permanent. "Patients can often achieve significant improvements in quality of life with minimal side effects, using very low doses of cannabinoids in the range of 10 mg to 60 mg per day," Sulak writes in his course materials: "A combination of THC, CBD, and other cannabinoids in various ratios can be used to fine-tune the benefits and minimize the side effects of cannabinoid treatment."Medical cannabis can help patients tolerate conventional cancer treatments like chemo and radiation, and can be used along with these treatments with a low likelihood of drug interaction. This means there is seldom a reason to avoid combining cannabis with conventional cancer treatments (with a few exceptions noted in the educational materials).

CANNABIS TO FIGHT CANCER AND PROMOTE HEALING

Along with symptom relief and improved quality of life in cancer patients, cannabinoids also have shown anticancer effects in many cell and animal experimental models. And a large body of anecdotal evidence suggests that human cancers also respond to cannabinoid treatment, Sulak observes. Several patients have reported slowing or arresting tumor growth, and others have experienced full remission of aggressive cancers while using cannabis extracts.To achieve these powerful anticancer effects, most patients need a higher dose than is needed for symptom relief — often 200 mg to 2,000 mg of cannabinoids a day, or the equivalent of one to two ounces of herbal cannabis a week. This treatment level may be cost effective if the cannabis is grown by a patient or caregiver outdoors, but purchasing this amount of medicine from a medical cannabis retailer could be expensive.At these high doses, Sulak says, "a knowledgeable medical provider must monitor the treatment to prevent side effects and interactions with conventional cancer treatment. Patients must carefully titrate up to reach these high doses without significant adverse effects. Surprisingly, doses in the range of 2,000 mg/day can be well tolerated."Any medical treatment carries certain risks, he adds, but high-dose cannabis is nonlethal and much safer than conventional chemotherapy, though the effectiveness of high-dose cannabis for cancer hasn't been studied in people. Some patients reaching very high doses report global improvement in symptoms and better quality of life. Others find that at ultrahigh doses the cannabis stops helping with symptoms like pain, anxiety, and sleep disturbance — benefits they easily achieved at lower doses. Still others fail to build tolerance to the adverse effects of high cannabis doses and find themselves stoned, groggy, and uncomfortable.

Choosing CBD products

CBD is a natural substance, but even natural substances must be approached with caution and due diligence. There's great variation in CBD products. Some CBD product labels make false health claims. In particular, CBD products purchased online have a high rate of mislabeling.After analyzing 84 CBD products sold online, researchers found that about 43 percent had a higher CBD concentration than stated. About 26 percent had less CBD than claimed. If you're

currently being treated for cancer,
keep in mind that many substances
can interact with other therapies.
That includes CBD, other
cannabinoids, or even dietary and
herbal supplements.

**Talk to your doctor about the
potential benefits and risks of
CBD, what to look for, and where
to purchase it. Here are a few
things to consider when choosing
CBD products:**

- Products with hemp-derived
  CBD should have only trace
  amounts of THC.

- Products with marijuana-
  derived CBD may contain
  enough THC to produce a high.
- Avoid products that make
  over-the-top health claims.
- Compare labels to see how
  much CBD is actually in the
  product.

It can take time to find the optimal
dose and feel the effects, so a little
patience is required. It's a good
idea to start with a small dose and
increase it gradually. You also want
to be sure to purchase a high-
quality CBD product from a
reputable company. Before buying,

research the company's reputation by reviewing its BBB ratings and seeing if it has received a warning letterTrusted Source from the FDA. The company should also offer a high level of transparency regarding the sourcing, manufacturing, and testing of its products.

Conclusion

CBD shouldn't be used in place of other cancer treatments. We need more rigorous studies into the potential benefits and risks of CBD, dosing, administration, and how it affects other cancer therapies.Currently, there are no FDA-approved CBD products for cancer. So, aside from Epidiolex for epilepsy, the products that are available haven't been evaluated by the FDA.Even so, some people are using cannabinoids to ease side effects of cancer treatment.

Because CBD can interact with other cancer therapies, it's best to check with your doctor before you start taking it.

Made in the USA
Middletown, DE
02 November 2023

41815012R00066